# ALS *meets* CHRIST

Life Lessons from
Surviving Lou Gehrig's
Disease since 2005

## CAROL FERGUSON

ALS MEETS CHRIST
Copyright © 2019 by Carol Ferguson

ISBN: 978-1-4866-1875-0
eBook ISBN: 978-1-4866-1901-6

Word Alive Press
119 De Baets Street Winnipeg, MB  R2J 3R9
www.wordalivepress.ca

WORD ALIVE
—P R E S S—

Cataloguing in Publication information can be obtained from Library and Archives Canada.

# Contents

# INTRODUCTION

God is the editor of my life. He decides the chapter headings, He adds a comma where I need to pause, and He corrects my errors by turning them into life lessons. I have given Him control of the story of my life, even this chapter called ALS.

Home is where your story begins. God is my home. He decided my DNA. He planted me in a family with Scottish and Norwegian roots, gave me blond hair, blue eyes, and a curious mind. He gave me a mother who taught me language skills, proper manners, and a sense of humour. He gave me a dad who modelled empathy, patience, a love of order, and who was a good example of a father. He gave me a sister, my sibling, role model, and the example I aspired to, who showed me what love is all about.

God has guided my life by whispers in my ear, nudges in my conscience, checks in my decisions, and His loving kindness when questions were unanswered. He gifted me with great faith in Him, the ability to take things to the cross and leave them there, and the belief that the answer would arrive in His time. Even in this journey through ALS, He has proved Himself faithful.

I do not have a degree in the medical profession, nor am I am trained as a Life Coach. So, you will not receive professional advice from me. However, as I write this book, I am entering my twelfth year since my own diagnosis with ALS.

In large part, I will deal with information you can find in "A Manual For People Living with ALS" (the "ALS Manual"), published by the ALS Society of Canada, or by researching online. However, in this book, I look at ALS from a Christian perspective. I have been a Christian much longer than I have had ALS. I trained in Christian Education at Winnipeg Bible College, now Providence Bible College, served for a dozen years as a missionary to Cree and Chipewyan people in Fort Chipewyan, Alberta, worked in several senior care homes, and ministered as Prayer Pastor/Pastor to seniors at Hillcrest Apostolic Church in Moose Jaw, Saskatchewan. All these things have shaped me into who I am today.

This book is different than most books about ALS because it includes things to do, books to read, scripture verses to memorize, and how to prepare for what the Lord has called you to, as well as some amazing things the Lord has taught me through my ALS journey. As 2 Corinthians says, "*Therefore we do not lose heart. Though outwardly we are wasting away, yet inwardly we are being renewed day by day*" (4:16, NLT).

CHAPTER ONE

# The Diagnosis

If you are reading this book, I assume you or someone you love is dealing with a diagnosis of Lou Gehrig's disease—ALS. Why is it called Lou Gehrig's disease? Lou was a great baseball player in the 1920–1930s, the first basemen with the Yankees through most of his baseball career. In fifteen years he accomplished 2,721 hits, 493 home runs, and 1,995 RBIs [Runs batted in]. He played with the New York Yankees in six World Series.

Then he began having physical problems and loss of strength, and, on his thirty-sixth birthday, he was diagnosed with Amyotrophic Lateral Sclerosis, ALS. On July 4, 1939, at the Lou Gehrig Appreciation Day at

Yankee Stadium, Lou spoke: "Fans, for the past two weeks you have heard about the bad break I got. Yet today I consider myself the luckiest man on the face of the earth. I've got a lot to live for."[1] He died two years later, leaving behind his wife, but no children. He set the bar high for a positive attitude towards ALS.

Doctors often hesitate to give harsh diagnoses like ALS, so you probably played what I call "the game" with several doctors, each one doing tests in their line of expertise.

I felt a lump in my throat, so my family doctor sent me to an Eye, Ear, Nose, and Throat specialist. After several tests, he told me that he didn't find a lump, but he added, "There is a name for that feeling: Globus Hystericus." I took that as a polite way to say I was hysterical. I really did feel a lump. Surprisingly, after I got the test results back, the lump was gone. I was referred to another doctor, who did an MRI of my brain.

Some people feel claustrophobic in that noisy, metal tube, being told to not move. I had trouble controlling my giggles. At one time, there were several loud knocks, like someone knocking on a door. Into my mind popped the song, "Knock Three Times" by Tony Orlando: "Oh, my darling, / knock three times on the ceiling if you need me, / twice on the pipes if the answer is 'No.'"

In 2005, a neurologist turned me into a human pin cushion, sticking needles into my muscles that were connected to a computer to record muscle activity.

---

[1] Steve Rotfeld Productions, "Greatest Sports Legends- Lou Gehrig's Farewell Speech" (video), published September 30, 2010, https://www.youtube.com/watch?v=626Dt9JdjQs&list=PL63TY5yYtZhQ1jscaaLHChBh-Xu60mCKK&index=47&t=0s.

There are no set rules to this game. It goes like this: the first doctor you see does tests in his line of expertise and recites a list of what the problem might be. The same thing happens with the next doctor and the next doctor, and on and on it goes, but with no diagnosis. Where does all this information end up? Who is actually in charge and gathering all this data together?

Meanwhile, the lists keep running through your mind, and eventually you become aware that ALS is on every list. By process of elimination, you ask the question: Is it ALS? It has been said that when everything else has been ruled out, it must be ALS.

Three little letters change your life forever: ALS or **A-myo-trophic-lateral-sclerosis**.

**A**bsence of >
**Myo** > Muscle
**Trophic** > Nourishment
**Lateral** > Side of (Spine)
**Sclerosis** >Hardening

The "ALS Manual" has long, medical explanations about chromosomes and motor neurons in the spinal cord and what areas of the body they control. But here is my uneducated explanation of ALS in a nut shell. *In the beginning, Zinc and Copper were happily married, living in our brain with their well-behaved muscle children. Then, in some brains, (and we don't know why), Zinc and Copper had a falling out, and they divorced. Each went their own way, both abdicating all responsibilities for their muscle children.*

*Neglected and undernourished, the muscle children eventually became weak, angry, and totally dysfunctional.*

Almost ten percent of people with ALS have what is called Familial ALS; it's inherited. Others have what is called Sporadic ALS, which means there is no known reason for it. ALS most commonly affects the lower limbs first, but, when it develops in the bulb area of the brain stem, it is called Bulbar ALS, and it affects the speaking and swallowing functions first. That type is said to progress the fastest. I have Sporadic Bulbar ALS.

After my diagnosis was confirmed, my doctor referred me to doctor at the ALS clinic at City Hospital in Saskatoon, Saskatchewan. My family doctor has been the steady hand in my situation. He listens to me. He is always one step ahead of me, like when he made sure I got a pneumonia shot and an annual flu shot. He is always encouraging and, like all my doctors, he is amazed I am still alive.

CHAPTER TWO

# Elephants in the Room

A n elephant in the room is a situation no one wants
to discuss or a condition no one wants to challenge.
There are several elephants stomping around in this ALS
enclosure. We'll call the first elephant *death*. Most of us do
not expect to face our own death, and so fear is often the
first response to a diagnosis of a terminal illness.

"Fear not" appears, in one form or another, 365 times
in the Bible, once for every day of the year. That should be
evidence that fear, which we can't turn off with the flick
of a switch, is always lying in wait. It also tells us that
the Lord knows and understands what we feel, and He is
prepared well ahead of time to meet our needs.

Everyone is destined to die, but we'd prefer to control the how, when, and where. If we could choose our moment of death, most of us would choose fast and painless. The one person who did have a choice, Jesus, did not choose fast or painless: "*He humbled himself and became obedient unto death, even the death of the cross*" (Philippians 2:8). He willingly went to the cross on our behalf.

1 John 4:18 tells us that "*Perfect love casteth out fear...*" and Christ's death on the cross was the result of perfect love. So, "*When I am afraid, I will put my trust in you, Lord. I praise God for what He has promised. I trust in God, so why should I be afraid?*" (Psalm 56:3–4, NLT). Burn those scriptures into your memory and quote them, yell them at the enemy, remind God of His promises, and use them to chase away fear.

There is another elephant in the room that you are probably face to face with right now. This elephant is a question: *Can God heal ALS?* There is only one answer for a Christian. Yes, He can. To say otherwise is to say that God is not our almighty, all powerful, omniscient God, the great I AM, and deny that Christ healed many when He lived here on earth. After my diagnoses with ALS, an elderly man in our church walked by me every Sunday after the service and softly said, "God made you, He can heal you."

One day Jesus and his disciples saw a blind man. The disciples asked Jesus, "*Master, who did sin, this man or his parents, that he was born blind?*" Jesus replied, "*Neither hath this man sinned nor his parents: but that the works of God should be made manifest Him*" (John 9:2–3).

Would the answer be different if they asked that question today? "Why does this person have ALS?" Or are you asking, "Why Me?" His answer is the same: *"that the works of God should be made manifest in you."*

That last statement is the one we need to focus on. Years ago, an elderly man lay dying. His granddaughter knew that he longed to see her committed to the Lord before he died. After her grandfather died, she came to our church seeking the Lord and found Him. She is still living for the Lord to this day. The Lord is always looking at the bigger picture.

There were multiple situations when Jesus healed people. Sometimes He healed everyone in the crowd, sometimes only one, or ten. But was there a reason for God's timing in any healing? The crippled man by the Pool of Bethesda had been there for thirty-eight years (John 5:5). The blind man had been blind since birth (John 9:1). Demons often threw a young boy into fire or water before Jesus healed him (Mark 9:22). Friends lowered a paralyzed man down through the roof to be near Jesus for healing (Mark 2:40).

They were all eventually healed by Jesus, but the timing of each one is unique. If the man had been waiting by the pool at Bethesda for only a month instead of thirty-eight years, would his healing have had such an impact? The blind man spent his entire life begging, long enough for everyone in the area to recognize him.

The last verse of the Faith Chapter says: *"All these people earned a good reputation because of their faith, yet none of them received all that God had promised. For God had something better in mind for us..."* (Hebrews 11:39–40, NLT).

Are you willing to wait for God's will to be made manifest in you, however long it takes? For the Lord to get the greater glory? George Mueller, a powerful man of God, stated: "Faith does not operate in the realm of the possible. There is no glory for God in that which is humanly possible. Faith begins where man's power ends."[2] Are you willing to die to bring that lost loved one to the Lord. Ask the Lord to heal you, but leave the decision to Him. He might have something better in mind.

I think we all agree that the Lord *can* heal ALS, but we don't know His time frame.

Our medical profession has put a timeline on ALS, usually two, five, or ten years. I have heard from missionaries in other countries that prayer is raising people from the dead; why is this not happening in ours? It may be that our society is so dependent on our medical system that we don't even ask God to heal. *It is time to change that!* If humanity has not found a cure for a disease, it is considered terminal. "Apart from God" is the key issue. I have heard of a couple of people who have been healed of ALS through prayer, however, the media is reluctant to share their stories. Pray for healing. Pray for courage. Pray for God to be glorified in and through you But, in all things, pray, *not my will, but thine be done.*

---

[2] The Famous People, "65 George Muller Quotes On God, Faith, Prayer And Humanity," https://quotes.thefamouspeople.com/george-muller-3815.php

## CHAPTER THREE
### *What Defines a Miracle?*

A miracle is an event that cannot be explained by natural or scientific laws. It is therefore a divine event. I want to share a story of a friend of mine, who had a degenerating heart. Her only hope was a heart transplant. She was single and alone facing this health problem. Our church, at that time, was studying Christ as our healer.

After much soul-searching and praying, she decided to ask the church board to pray for her healing, as James 5:14–16 teaches. Some board members admitted that they did not expect God to heal her, but they anointed her with oil and prayed for her anyway.

Her next medical check-up was on a Wednesday—prayer meeting night. That evening she phoned the church to tell everyone that after nine hours of medical tests, the doctors said she had the heart of a newborn baby. For those who question this, it is all documented in her medical records. I saw her years later, still thriving. As the song "My God is So Big" by Ruth Harms Calkin says, "My God is so big, / so strong and so mighty, / there's nothing my God cannot do."

If you are a pessimist, and you don't believe in miracles, you need to know that pessimism is a learned condition. Otherwise, there would not be so many scriptures telling us how to change our mind: "*Be not conformed to this world: but ye be transformed by the renewing of your mind, that you may prove what is that good, and acceptable, and perfect will of God*" (Romans 12:2). Retraining your brain isn't a simple task, and it takes determination and dedication, but it can be done.

We see miracles all the time, but don't recognize them as such. How about that town drunk, the one you crossed the street to avoid, who gave his life to Jesus, quit drinking, and became an important part of the community? Or how about that kid from a dysfunctional home, who became a child of God, and with His help, made it through college and started his own business? Every salvation story is a miracle. Miracles even happen in the surgical ward, astonishing doctors.

Do you need to retrain your brain? Philippians 4:8 says, "*Finally, brethren, whatsoever things are true,* *whatsoever things are honorable, whatsoever things are just, whatsoever things are pure, whatsoever things are lovely, whatsoever things are of good report… <u>think on these things</u>"* (emphasis added). Then read verse seven: "*And the peace of God, which passeth all understanding, will keep your hearts and your <u>minds</u> through Christ Jesus*" (emphasis added). Miracles surpass all understanding. Change your mind and you'll see miracles.

Read up on what God is doing in other countries. God has gifted our medical personnel with extraordinary wisdom, just like he gifted people in the Old Testament to build the tabernacle, the temple, and the ark. Find and read true stories, such as *Ninety Minutes in Heaven*, by Don Piper, about people who have been healed or delivered.

The Serenity Prayer, by Reinhold Niebuhr, contains all we need from the Lord: "God, grant me the serenity to accept the things I cannot change, courage to change the things I can, and wisdom to know the difference."

## CHAPTER FOUR
# A Cross of Victory

It's been said that a diagnosis can be a blessing or a curse. Many people, having been diagnosed with ALS, respond in anger, sit down, and wait to die. Then it does become a curse. But Jesus said, in Mark 8:34, "...*Whosoever will come after me, let him deny himself, and take up his cross, and follow me.*"

We have lost sight of what a cross is. It isn't a job I don't like, or my financial situation, or something that bugs me. Something that I whine and groan about is not a cross I have to bear, but "a chip on the shoulder." To pick up the cross is to die to self and put Christ first.

Christ did not view the cross as a negative thing. It became His place of victory, where He died, paid the price for our sin, and then rose victorious, the greatest miracle

Scripture tells us in Matthew 5:23–25 that if we have anything against someone, we should make it right. Likewise, if we know anyone who has something against us, we need to make it right. Does that seem fair to you, that either way, it's up to you? Ask the Lord to show you if there are things you need to say, and to whom. Here are a few ideas.

*I love you.* In some families this is tossed about flippantly. If it isn't part of your vocabulary, it should be. Say "I love you" with feeling to someone, and you might hear, "I love you, too."

*I was wrong.* Certain people never say, "I'm sorry," because nothing is ever their fault. I once heard this quote, and it has stuck with me ever since: "The person most likely to be deceitful is the one who is under the most pressure to succeed." If you have been putting the pressure on someone about a job, education, or life style, say "I'm Sorry," and set them free. If you're the one who is under pressure to please someone or do something, give it to the Lord. He will help you with your burden. He loves you, and He is pleased with you.

*Forgive me.* Forgiving and being forgiven is often misunderstood. The Lord's prayer, *"and forgive us our sins, as we have forgiven those who sin against us"* (Matthew 6:12, NLT), deals with both aspects. In medical books, unforgiveness is classified as a disease, according a doctor at the Cancer Treatment Centers of America. An often-used quote says, "Not forgiving is like drinking acid and expecting the other person to die."[3] No matter who is at fault, you take the initiative and say "Forgive Me!" Let the Lord deal with the outcome. That's His business.

*I'm proud of you.* God said it at Jesus' baptism in Matthew 3:17: "...*This is my beloved son, in whom I am well pleased.*" Many people go through life without ever feeling appreciated. That's sad, but love and appreciation from God are even more important than from people. ALS puts a lot of pressure on the family. If you are the one who is never grateful, it's time to change that and start thanking people for everything they do for you.

This is your opportunity change "a chip on the shoulder" into a cross of victory.

---

[3] The origins of this quote are not clear. Alan Brandt was quoted in print in 1995 as saying "Being resentful, they say, is like taking poison and waiting for the other person to die." Others attribute this quote to Nelson Mandela.

CHAPTER FIVE

## Leave a Legacy

People leave different kinds of legacies when they die. Financial legacies might be the most common, but not always the most beneficial (the difference between giving a man a fish, or teaching him how to fish).

You might have inherited your intelligence, sense of humour, compassion, or work ethic from parents and grandparents, and you will pass those on to your family, too. But there are other details you need to take care of to prepare your family, like updating your will, naming a Power of Attorney, and making funeral arrangements. Make a decision about a DNR [do not resuscitate] directive. Update your medication list. Make a list of passwords you use, how to access a safety deposit box, and where you have hidden things.

My great-grandfather fought in the Civil War. Years later, his children found his weapons and played with them. My great-grandmother was so upset that she buried them in the back yard and never told anyone where. Our legacy is buried somewhere.

How many times have you heard people say they wished they had asked more questions before a friend or loved one died? Ask your family what things they want to hear about and have fun working on memories together. Write about crazy things you did and laugh together. Write about family holidays, even one page per event, will do. Write about family traditions when you were little. Memories are part of your legacy, too.

The most important legacy is a spiritual legacy. Make sure family and friends know about your spiritual journey. If you have young people in the family who are going the wrong way, they need to hear about the times you goofed up.

This is a good time to write a letter to a special friend or a teacher who made a difference in your life. There may be people who are not aware that the Lord has changed your life, and there certainly are people who would want to be praying for you as you deal with ALS.

Perhaps you have sung the hymn, "Take My Life and Let it Be" by Frances Ridley Havergal:

Take my life and let it be
consecrated, Lord, to thee;

....

Take my hands and let them move
at the impulse of Thy love.
Take my feet and let them be
swift and beautiful for thee.
Take my voice and let me sing,
always, only, for my King.

You probably never imagined that, someday, ALS would show up and take away all those options. Are you willing to give the Lord total control of your life, hands, feet, and voice? When does ALS meet Christ? The moment you take up your cross and decide to willingly follow Christ through the valley called ALS.

There are certain emotional states we go through in dealing with a terminal illness, whether you, a friend, or a loved one is dying. The important thing is to allow the Lord to walk with you through every emotion. The Lord won't mind if you yell at Him and tell Him you don't want to go through this. Loneliness isn't reserved for after a loved one dies. Loneliness takes place whenever you are apart.

Everyone deals differently and for varied lengths of time with grief. You might feel shock, guilt, anger, disbelief, or numbness, and any one of those can bring about physical pain, headaches or stomach aches. Get medical or emotional help if necessary.

Some families have a great sense of humour that turns every difficulty into a blessing. Another families may be pessimistic and see nothing positive in anything. Some may deny the truth. Some people share everything, and other people bury their feelings deep inside and refuse to even tell a loved one they have ALS. Once ALS is diagnosed, you will need to talk this through. When the time is right, talk to the children in your life, too. They don't always understand what they "overheard." They need to know the truth, even if it is painful. Talk to them about heaven and the process of dying. Talk through questions.

We'll talk more about end of life care further on in the book. Now might be a good time to think ahead, maybe talk about the need to move to another location in the future. I decided to sell my house and move while I still had the strength to be a part of the packing, sorting, and blessing friends and family with meaningful items.

Now take some time to be a little selfish. Have you seen the movie *The Bucket List?* It is the story of two eccentric men, both facing death, who share a hospital room. Over the course of time, they decide to go away together and do the things they always wanted to do, before they "Kicked the Bucket." They made their bucket list. You can make a bucket list and add it to your legacy.

Your list might be as simple as visiting the old homestead once more, or it may be a desire to see the ocean or the mountains for the first time, go sky diving, or to take a trip to Europe. (Don't leave home without a medic alert bracelet on your wrist.) I moved into a seniors' high rise and then I went on a short cruise with some of the family. I took a helicopter trip to the top of a glacier with my sister, which was a great time of bonding.

We let the cruise line know ahead of time that I had eating problems, and they provided me with my own personal waiter. He presented me with a meal of things I could eat three times a day. Note: if you decide to fly somewhere, be aware of what you can and can't take on an airplane. You can't take unopened bottles of Ensure on a plane, but you may be able take along dry pudding mix or instant breakfast to add to beverages purchased after going through customs. If you decide to go on a road trip, you can make arrangements to refill oxygen tanks along the way.

Maybe you want to see the ballet or a concert. This might be a good time to have a family reunion. My mother took swimming lessons when she was in her seventies. Make a bucket list, no matter how ridiculous some of the ideas are. Do what you can. Have fun!

CHAPTER SIX

# How Would You Handle Healing?

When I was diagnosed, there were seven people living in Moose Jaw with ALS. All my friends, family, and church who prayed for me, were a great blessing, but a strange thing took place in my mind about them. Once, as people were praying for my healing, I thought, *they shouldn't be praying for me. When I die, I'll go to heaven. They should be praying for people with ALS who don't know the Lord.* Thus began my journey of guilt. Isaiah 42:8 says, *"I am the Lord; that is my name: and my glory I will not give to another..."* So, I resisted healing.

I have read stories where hundreds of people met in the church basement to pray for revival, and when it came, they all quit praying to join the rejoicing upstairs. I have heard of two people healed from ALS as a result of prayer. I have seen God do amazing things in the past, but I have also seen a church or a person take the glory when someone was healed. It is easy for a miracle to turn into a sensation. As silly as it sounds, I feared being healed. I was afraid that if I was healed I would become proud and God would not get all the glory. I was afraid too, that our city or church would become a destination for others looking for healing. I remember praying, "Lord, keep me in the basement praying."

But I still continued to ask for prayer for healing. I even flew to Toronto to attend a conference at the Toronto Airport Church, well known for its healing ministry. At the next visit to my ALS doctor, he took a long time checking me over and re-reading my file. Finally, he stated, almost under his breath, "This is benign." I didn't know how to handle that. It's hard to tell people that the Lord has done something amazing when nothing has changed.

Over the course of a few years, one by one, every other person with ALS in Moose Jaw died. I attended the funeral of one that I had known quite well, and I felt enormous guilt— Survivor's guilt. I felt I should have done something, when though there was nothing I could do.

Eventually, God did a new thing in my heart, and I felt I would be able to deal with my own healing. I realized my life was in His hands, and I knew He had a reason. However, most of all I want God to receive the greater glory, no matter what that means for me.

## CHAPTER SEVEN

# What About Your Medical Team?

Now, let's get down to actually dealing with ALS. It's becoming the norm for people to take more control of their own medical treatment. If your family doctor has little experience with ALS or none at all, he/she should be willing to refer you to another doctor who has dealt with ALS before. You have a right to ask to be referred to a specialist. A neurologist will make the final diagnosis, which will probably include an MRI [magnetic resonance imaging] to take pictures of your brain activity, and an EMG [electromyogram], where a needle is inserted into various muscles so that a computer can read muscle activity.

A specialist may put you on Rilutek, an ALS medication made and distributed from Quebec. Not everyone with ALS can tolerate Rilutek because it can affect the kidneys, but regular blood test will keep an eye on that.

Rilutek is expensive, so check to see what help is available to cover the cost. There is a benevolent plan for those over sixty-five. Rilutek is not available from a pharmacist, but can be ordered through your ALS clinic.

Your ALS Society is part of your team too. Comprised of people who have ALS, their family and friends, or those who have lost someone to ALS, they understand what you are going through.

Every province has an ALS Society (the North West Territories, the Yukon, and Nunavut are each included with a province). Find the ALS Society nearest to you, get involved, and ask questions. They will give you "A Manual For People Living with ALS," which explains issues people with ALS face, where you can go for support, and tips for coping. They keep up with available treatment and equipment. They will also be able to tell you what programs and equipment are available. Check out what your Society can provide for you, such as funding a ramp for your house, a suction machine to use at home, braces, and appliances to help you grip or reach things. They will do whatever they can to assist you in your daily living, even provide a LINK computer to talk on the telephone for you. They can put you in touch with the nearest Aids for Independent Living program. In some provinces, the Red Cross looks after that, but others have their own outlet.

The ALS Society also hosts fund raisers. I take part in the annual Walk for ALS, and I will for as long as I can. ALS walks are laid out so people can walk for as long as their strength allows. If you can't walk, then get a friend or family member to push you in a wheelchair. Many people with ALS even take part in marathons, using an adult jogging stroller.

My first ALS walk was only six kilometres, when I still had lots of strength. Several years later, I took part in Kim's Walk for ALS, hosted by Kim Dolinski annually for her dad, who has ALS. It's a twenty-four-kilometre walk from Regina to Lumsden, Saskatchewan. Kim walks it every year, even if she is alone.

I spent months on a treadmill and the Rotary Club walking trails in Moose Jaw, preparing for Kim's Walk. My family also took part, two walking, two biking, one hauling supplies, and giving moral support. It took me four hours and fifteen minutes, and I met a lot of new friends. I made it to the end, exhausted, with blisters on blisters. That was a once-in-a-lifetime accomplishment.

CHAPTER EIGHT
## On Being Speechless

I'm going to avoid all tongue in cheek statements people make about a woman who can't talk. When I was diagnosed with Bulbar ALS and started to lose my speech, I worked with seniors, visiting at the hospital and seniors' homes. As my speech got worse, it became evident that, with my poor speech and so many seniors hard of hearing, I would have to resign.

My life became a constant game of charades as friends tried to interpret what I was trying to say. I started out using a whiteboard and dry erase markers. It always makes me laugh when people forget that I can't talk. One day, some friends and I were talking about speaking more than one language. I told them (wrote on my slate) that I learned to speak Cree when I lived in the north.

"Say something for us in Cree," one of them suggested. There was total silence. Then everyone burst out laughing. That said to me that being speechless is no big deal and life goes on. I taunt friends with the fact that I can "talk" in church and they can't. But on the other hand, I can't talk in the dark, or visit with my blind friends.

One of my great-granddaughters kept her distance from me, almost as if she was afraid of me. Someone must have talked to her because one day she said to me, "You can't talk, can you?" I shook my head no and she threw herself into my arms and hugged me.

The "ALS Manual" states that the loss of speech may be the end of off-the-cuff remarks. Not so! I enjoy writing teasing comments to the teenagers and young adults in my extended family. Finally, one of them jokingly told me, "You'd better be quiet or we'll take your board away from you." That's a threat I hear often.

I graduated from the whiteboard to the Boogie Board eWriter tablet, which you write on with a stylus (or your fingernail), with a battery-operated eraser, good for 50,000 erases. (It was also the highest selling toy in 2012). Kids love it and it is a great ice breaker, even with children who can't read. You can draw pictures for them, or let them scribble on it. Today's children are used to laptops and cell phones. Even a baby will enjoy pushing the button to erase what you've drawn. The next step will be a talking iPad.

Our society has lost the ability to be silent, but it has also blessed us with a myriad of ways to communicate. Being unable to use a telephone might not be due to loss of speech, but the inability to lift the receiver. There is a hands free-phone that is activated by blowing on a switch, along with an operator dialing system.

Email might be your choice, rather than the telephone. There are computers that can speak what you type and/or read for you. Facebook is a great way to stay connected with family and friends. Using Facebook to encourage others who have ALS has been a ministry for me at times.

While there are many methods for communicating without speech, some people prefer not to use tech. It is your choice, but talk it over with your family or caregivers, and keep in mind how long you will be able to use a certain device. Many ALS authors have written their biographies one letter at a time with a laser light, and more are being written all the time. You can find some of those books on Amazon, like *Eric Is Winning!!* by Eric Edney, *Cries of the Silent* by Evelyn Bell, and *The Luckiest Man: The Life and Death of Lou Gehrig* by Jonathan Eig.

Developing technology to help with communication is an ever-widening field. Most computer systems can be updated from hand use to a laser beam operated by head movement, eye blinks, or another part of the body, even your nose, to point to letters on a communication board. The Speech/Language pathologist at your ALS clinic will walk you through what's available. Word prediction is already in use on your cell phone, listing possible words after the first two letters are typed. Abbreviations and acronyms, like "R U OK?," are commonplace and make writing easier. These methods may not be faster, however; using retinal recognition can take up to forty-five minutes to write a sentence.

Most of this technology is expensive, but you may be able to find it second-hand.

## CHAPTER NINE
### *Things That Surprised Me*

Many things surprised me as I dealt with ALS. How it affects emotions caught me totally off guard. With some people, it shows up in the form of uncontrollable weeping, while others get uncontrollable laughter. *I got the laughter.* I have always laughed a lot, so it wasn't noticeable at first. My family and friends have learned to be careful when they make a funny remark. If I am taking a drink, I choke. Or if I am eating and have my mouth full, people are in grave danger of being sprayed. It took one embarrassing situation before I realized ALS caused this.

I went on a trip with family members, and, at one point, I started laughing for no reason. I couldn't stop.

My sister thought I was laughing at her, and I couldn't even catch my breath to explain. It caused hurt feelings until I could control myself and explain what happened. We hugged and cried together, and all was well again. It's something to be aware of. I'm glad I got the laughter and not uncontrollable weeping.

• • •

Obviously, whoever came up with the word "phlegm" did not take phonics in school. Maybe the same person came up with "phone," "phobia," and "phooey." Anyway, however it's spelled, it surprised me. Phlegm, or post nasal drip, is annoying when you have trouble swallowing. A lot of things that slide down your throat easily, like ice cream and milk, add to the build-up of phlegm. Then I heard that papaya enzymes could help. I tried it and it worked. I buy chewable papaya enzyme tablets and grind them in my coffee grinder. I always have some on hand, and when needed, I put a small amount at a time in my mouth. As it dissolves, it takes away the phlegm. Be careful not to breathe in the powder. Other suggestions are meat tenderizer mixed with a little water, or an expectorant cough syrup.

• • •

I had no idea that ALS affects your skin. Our skin is the largest and fastest growing organ in our body. Skin is your body's coat. It helps you stay warm, or cools you off, and it keeps germs out.

I became aware of changes in my skin when I noticed dandruff flaking off every part of my body and discovered my arms were scaly. Then I heard several friends talk about "dry brushing," which sounded like something that could help my situation. Dry brushing is exactly what it sounds like—brushing the skin in a particular pattern with a dry brush. Some people use it to stimulate blood flow or the lymph system, but my only reason is to cleanse and moisturize my skin.

Choose a firm, natural bristle brush with a long handle to allow you to reach your entire back, the bottoms of the feet, and backs of the legs. Don't brush too hard; your skin should never turn red or sting. Doing this in an empty bathtub makes it easy to clean up the blizzard of dander. You can stand or sit on a bath chair. Start at your feet and work up, brushing your skin with the brush, dry, no water. Brushing toward the heart is said to promote circulation. When you finish brushing, you are already in place to shower and apply a moisturizing lotion. My choice is coconut oil.

The change in your skin may be an annoyance that comes with the ALS, but it also brings with it a great blessing. Mesenchymal stem cell use is the use of a patient's own stem cells for healing. Did you know that stem cells can be harvested from your own dermis to be used in your fight against ALS? This avoids the ethical debate about embryonic stems cell use.

Using one's own stem cells can slow down the ALS symptoms and prolong life. There are no side effects and no risk of rejection. There are fewer fasciculations [brief, spontaneous contractions affecting a small number of muscle fibres, often causing a flicker of movement under the skin]; reflexes become more normal, limb movement increases, and swallowing and speech improves. ALS stem cell therapy opens new possibilities in treatment.

In European clinics, this therapy is considered the most modern and effective treatment for ALS. Clinical trials have proved it is safe, but the data was not recorded or has not been shared. Neither Health Canada or U.S. Food and Drug Administration have approved funding for this research. So, let's not complain about the dandruff flaking off our skin. It just could save our lives.

• • •

The Ice Bucket Challenge in Canada raised $17 million due to the generosity of more than 260,000 Canadians. The ALS Societies invested $10 million in ALS research and $7 million in programs that deliver critical support to Canadians living with ALS. The funds for ALS were matched on a one-to-one basis through a new research partnership with Brain Canada, bringing the total investment in ALS research to $20 million, the largest one-time investment in the ALS Canada Research Program in history.

Thank you to the people who started the Ice Bucket Challenge. Chris Kennedy, a professional golfer, challenged his sister, Jeanette Senerchia, whose husband, Anthony has ALS. A Facebook friend connected to a friend, who connected to a friend, and on and on it went. The Ice Bucket Challenge has levelled the financial field to a great extent. Suddenly, ALS has a platform for raising funds and it has been a huge success.

It used to bother me to see stores stocked with a multitude of items to raise awareness for cancer, the Heart and Stroke Foundation, Multiple Sclerosis, and other diseases. Then I realized it's because those diseases have many survivors. Few ALS patients live beyond ten years.

I took part in the challenge on my seventy-fifth birthday. Four generations of my family took part. I gave my son permission to pour a small bucket of ice water on my head. Behind my back, he switched the small bucket for a five-gallon pail (my family always has fun). It was a shock when five gallons of ice and water poured over my head, but the family was prepared with towels and blankets to warm me up quickly. Just another thing that surprised me. Would I do it again? Yes! Two of my great-grand-children took part in that challenge with me. My great-grandson, five years old at the time, stole the day. Standing on the sidewalk, shivering, teeth chattering, he stated, "I thought it was going to be warm." Somehow, he missed the word "ice" in the Ice Bucket Challenge.

# CHAPTER TEN
## *More Surprises*

I kept asking people if ALS includes pain, but no one ever answered me. I found out on my own that there is pain, usually from muscle cramps. A cramp can turn a hand into a claw, and cramps in the feet or legs are excruciating. Even healthy football players roll on the ground when their leg cramps. Walking can alleviate them, but if you can't get up on your feet to walk, something else is needed. Cramps are often caused by a lack of calcium or liquids, so liquid calcium is the answer. I take that at bedtime. Dairy products, dark leafy greens, and broccoli are also high in calcium.

I get cramps in my ribs if I bend a certain way, cramps in my neck if I twist the wrong way, and cramps in my hands when I'm trying to open a jar. There are electric gadgets now that will open jars. I have also switched to an electric can opener, and I have pliers in my silverware drawer. Some things have to wait until someone stronger visits.

• • •

Another symptom of ALS that was a surprise to me is jumping muscles, as opposed to muscle spasms or cramps. They don't hurt. They are just annoying and are actually visible when the muscles start to jump. I call them Mexican Jumping Beans. I started early on to give them to the Lord. When a muscle began to jump, I would put my hand over it, and ask the Lord to take it away. I have no scriptural backing for that. I guess the Lord nudged me because, eventually, they disappeared. That might not work for everyone, but I'm always ready to ask the Lord for help.

• • •

Changes quickly began to take place in my mouth and tongue, and people asked if I had new dentures. I had all my own teeth, but there was something wrong with my speech. I soon couldn't stick out my tongue, blow out a candle, or pucker my lips to whistle, the result of Bulbar ALS. My tongue now looks like "road kill" and pushes food out of my mouth, like a baby. So, I eat, I put food into my mouth and hold it shut with a paper towel until I swallow. I do the same thing when I drink.

I have to use thin-rimmed glasses or cups, but nothing with a thick rim. I have to make sure my tongue is in the right place before I swallow. I jokingly say that if I get a good siphoning action going I can swallow several times in a row. Thicken Up is a powder that thickens liquids to help with swallowing and is available at many pharmacies.

Your tongue is a voluntary muscle, so with ALS you don't automatically swallow your saliva; it just runs out of your mouth unless you concentrate on swallowing. There are mouth sprays for dry mouth, a common outcome of drooling.

Some people use washable cloths for wiping their mouths when they drool, but I prefer paper towels, which I call "diapers for my mouth." I have found a brand that works well for me and I have a constant supply folded and available by my chair, my bed, my desk, and even in my car. Like a person with a constant runny nose, I make sure I have somewhere to discard all those paper towels (Doggie Doo Doo bags are a perfect size). I am often asked if I had just had a dental work done.

Anti-nausea pills or patches, used for motion sickness, lessen saliva. I don't drool when I'm sleeping, which, I'm told, is typical of a mouth breather. I am blessed. I have the Lord to thank for helping me deal with the embarrassment of drooling. Once, at a football game, I saw 30,000 football fans spitting sunflower shells on the floor of the stands. ALS Drooling is not *that* gross.

## CHAPTER ELEVEN
## *Inhale and Exhale*

I had asthma as I child, so I'm used to minor breathing problems, but ALS has its own challenges. Several times, I have had a bad cough that needed to be cleared up with antibiotics and the help of a nebulizer; SAIL [Saskatchewan Aids for Independent Living] provided me with one to have at home from. My normal breathing has always been shallow—I inhale more than I exhale—but it has seldom restricted what I could do.

My choir director at Bible college explained how to breathe properly using your diaphragm. I have started to use my diaphragm again, exhaling harder and longer. Even now, when my lungs start to get a bit "wheezy," I make an extra effort to breathe out as hard as I can. If you need help coughing, it has been suggested that you put your fists on your abdomen and press up as you cough, as if you were doing the Heimlich manuever.

I am including the following information, *only* because pacing for the diaphragm [the rhythmic application of electrical impulses to the diaphragm to provide support for respiratory failure] is being researched and is worth keeping tabs on. In the 1950s, they used phrenic (diaphragm) nerve stimulation to treat patients with polio, with little success.

During the polio epidemic in Manitoba in the 1950s, I went to King George Hospital in Winnipeg, now the Riverview Health Centre, to visit a friend. There are some similarities between ALS and polio, but with polio, involuntary muscles, like the lungs, can be affected, and the onset is sudden. I saw patients, immobile on their backs, in a huge metal tube (an iron lung), with only their heads visible. Their minds were clear, and they could communicate with visitors. I am glad I went to visit her. I watched as a nurse hooked her up to a machine that coughed for her, a learning experience for me.

It would be thirty or forty years before anything more was developed for the diaphragm, when physicians experimented with nerve stimulation to produce contraction of the diaphragm. Current systems involve an external transmitter and an implanted receiver. Due to an inability to synchronize "diaphragmatic pacing" with natural breathing for patients with ALS in respiratory failure, the trial was stopped. Fully implantable diaphragmatic pacing systems are still in the works.

Noninvasive ventilation (such as what is used for sleep apnea) is part of the standard of care for treatment of respiratory failure in patients with ALS. Some other means of supporting respiratory function are more appealing to ALS patients.

Seven ALS centres in the U.K. conducted a DiPALS [Diaphragm pacing] study[4] with seventy-four patients, who were divided between noninvasive ventilation alone or that plus diaphragm pacing. They discovered survival was shorter when both were used together. Research has also shown that there is a progression of ALS after any surgical procedure.

---

[4] DiPALS Writing Committee, "Safety and efficacy of diaphragm pacing in patients with respiratory insufficiency due to amyotrophic lateral sclerosis (DiPALS): a multicentre, open-label, randomised controlled trial," *The Lancet Neurology* 14, no. 9 (Fall 2015): 883–892, https://www.thelancet.com/journals/laneur/article/PIIS1474-4422(15)00152-0/fulltext.

CHAPTER TWELVE

## Oral Health

Brushing your teeth is something we've been taught to do from early childhood, and we take it for granted. It isn't an easy task if you are losing muscle strength in your hands or if you have Bular ALS. Muscles in your mouth tend to have a mind of their own and will clamp down on the toothbrush without warning. If it's an electric toothbrush, that will "rattle your brain." However, an electric toothbrush is the best choice if you have weakened muscles in your hands.

Dental appointments can be a fearful event: fear that water will run down your throat and cause you to choke; fear that excess mucus will clog your breathing when you're tipped way back in the chair. Make arrangements to have the same dental hygienist at every appointment so they are aware of your fears.

One suggestion ALS patients hear is that you should get all your old amalgam fillings replaced because they contain mercury. Research has proved that amalgam fillings are not to blame for many of the diseases that people associate them with. A dental checkup will reveal if there is a problem with those old fillings, or, if one of them is leaking, then your dentist will probably advise having it removed.

Are you aware that dentists hate to pull a tooth? After all, a tooth pulled eliminates all future revenue from said tooth. Take control. They are your teeth. I used to bite my cheek whenever I sneezed, and often at night, which disrupted my sleep. I pinned the problem down to one molar and asked the dentist to pull it out. He refused.

After a few more weeks, I went back and demanded that the tooth be pulled. I had to do some fast talking (writing) to explain: since I couldn't chew, the molar was useless anyway. Reluctantly, they extracted the tooth. Problem solved and I sneeze in comfort.

I like the statement: Focus on what you can do rather than on what you can't do. I once saw a video of Stephen Hawking celebrating a milestone.[5] He depended on technology for everything. When the host proposed a toast, someone dripped a few drops of champagne on his tongue. Do what you can for as long as you can. I raise my

[5] Discovery U.K., "The Best of Stephen Hawking" (video), published March 18, 2018, https://www.youtube.com/watch?v=vkPn-Mbk3MA.

hands in worship during church services. I have done that for years. There might come a time when I can't do that, but I will for as long as I can. After all, praise is all about the Lord. One of Hawking's famous quotes is: "I have noticed even people who claim everything is predestined, and that we can do nothing to change it, look before they cross the road."[6]

---

[6] Stephen Hawking, "Is Everything Determined," *Black Holes and Baby Universes and Other Essays* (New York, NY: Bantam Books, 1993).

## CHAPTER THIRTEEN
### The Feeding Tube

Two of my doctors felt I should have a feeding tube put in, mainly in preparation for when I would need it. At that time, it was my tenth year with ALS, and I was cooking and eating well by mouth. Consider a feeding tube if you are losing weight, if it takes you more than an hour to eat a meal, or if you choke often. There are a couple types of PEG [percutaneous endoscopic gastrostomy] procedures, in which a tube is surgically inserted through the wall of the stomach for long-term external nutrition. Talk to people who rely on feeding tubes for nutrition for more information, or health care workers who have experience in that area.

Some feeding tubes, usually those for children, are held in place with a balloon and can easily be replaced at home, even by a child. Mine is an eight-inch external tube that can only be removed or replaced surgically. Inserting the tube was day surgery, and I went home that afternoon. Never having had surgery before, I discovered that every muscle in your body is connected to the stomach muscles. I was in pain.

There is a procedure to stretch the throat to make swallowing easier, if your doctor is willing. It surprised me to discover that, since they put in my feeding tube, I swallow better. My doctor said he didn't intentionally stretch my throat, so the tube used during surgery must have done the job. I only use my feeding tube for getting extra liquids into my system. Lately, I have learned that concentrated juices, which taste good and slide down well, contain very little water, and so are not a good choice.

Depending on where the tube is placed, you might have to make some changes in clothing. I am short and also have a short torso, so my tube is pretty well at waist level. Most of my slacks have elastic waists or Velcro fastening. The alternative is to have a nasal tube surgically installed (nasogastric intubation), which runs through your nose into your stomach. You can find lots of good videos online about tube feeding.

There are two ways to deliver a tube feeding. One is gravity feeding, where the bag is hung on an IV pole and flows into the tube, or a feeding pump may be used. Portable pumps are available, and, once you are getting all your nutrition via tube feedings, home care provides your nutrition.

The main problem I have with my tube is leakage around the tube, which leads to a problem with granulated flesh. Home care nurses come to visit me weekly to keep an eye on it, and they provide dressings and swabs. They also do Silver Nitrate treatments as needed to burn away granulated tissue, but that has to be applied two or three days in a row to be effective.

I've been on a journey learning to deal with granulated flesh. Sugar and honey have treated battle wounds for thousands of years. When my grandmother suffered with leg ulcers, they didn't respond to any medication, so the hospital staff resorted to packing the ulcers with sugar and adding a dressing. Sugar adds oxygen to the area and ulcers are usually caused by poor circulation. It worked for her.

Bees use an enzyme known as glucose oxidase in making honey. That enzyme breaks down the glucose to make hydrogen peroxide and that makes honey a natural antiseptic. I found Manuka honey in a health food store, which is made from bees using Manuka plant pollen. I clean my stoma (a Greek word meaning "opening," referring to the surgical site where the tube is installed), smear on the honey, and cover it with a dressing. It is very soothing. I never eat honey; it is sticky and causes choking.

Then I discovered something even better. I bought an aloe plant and started using fresh aloe oil. It has cleared up most of the granulated tissue and there is much less leaking. Maalox or Dioval can also be used on irritated skin in the stoma area.

## CHAPTER FOURTEEN
### How Much does Your Head Weigh?

I began having problems with weak neck muscles, mostly when out walking. I couldn't hold my head up straight because it felt so heavy, and soon it became painful. I bought a sponge neck brace, but being soft, it only helped to a certain extent. I even made a classy cover to put over it, or, if I was wearing a turtleneck shirt, I wrapped the collar up around the foam.

Why don't neck muscles get tired and sore when you are sitting? When you walk, you glance down at the path. Sitting, you look ahead. How much does a head weigh, anyway? It's impossible to weigh your head on a scale; I tried it so I know. You can't read the weight with your head on the scale. A Google search told me that ten pounds is the average weight of a head. Now we realize how important our neck muscles are in keeping the head balanced upright. Your doctor will caution you; that the more you depend on a neck brace the less work your own muscles do.

A physical therapy centre can give you exercises for your neck. They involve turning, twisting, and bending the head and upper body, and doing isometric exercises. The isometric neck stretch is one of the best ways to give your neck muscles the exercise they need. You can do them anywhere, even out in public, and they build endurance, power, and flexibility in the neck muscles. Place both your palms on your forehead. Push your head forward while resisting with your palms. Hold for five to eight seconds and repeat three times.

Next, put your hands behind your head, pushing and resisting for five to eight seconds and repeat three times. Do the same thing on each side of your head, pushing with your head, resisting with your palm. The plank, side plank, and the wall sit are also isometric exercises. You can find more information if you Google exercises for neck muscles.

A bent neck or a humped back could be the result of sleeping with too many pillows or using a walker that is not correctly adjusted to your height. I did away with my usual pillows and now sleep with only one, a bone shaped, neck support pillow. It is much easier on my neck.

The Headmaster Collar is the neck brace I use now. It is rigid and was adjusted to fit me at the Wascana

Rehabilitation Centre in Regina. It allows enough movement to shoulder check when driving. I take it off at home and when my neck begins to ache.

## CHAPTER FIFTEEN
### *Revealed and Glorified*

A friend complained one day on his way to yet another chemotherapy treatment for cancer. "I don't want to go there," he told the Lord. "It isn't even helping." Then, the Lord spoke to him, saying, "No, but *I* want to be there." With a diagnosis of ALS, you have the divine opportunity to take Christ to places where you may not want to go, but where Christ wants to be: "...*Christ in you, the hope of glory*" (Colossians 1:27).

Did you know the Bible tells us we will glorify God when we die from ALS?

Jesus said to Peter, in John 21:18, NLT: "...*When you were young, you were able to do as you liked; you dressed yourself and went wherever you wanted to go. But when you are old, you will stretch out your hands, and others will dress you and take you where you don't want to go."* That sounds like the road ahead for those of us with ALS. However, verse 19 tells us: *"Jesus said this to let him [Peter] know by what kind of death he [Peter] would glorify God..."* When not a single muscle is working, and you can't do anything physical, you can still glorify the Lord. You can still carry on a vibrant prayer ministry.

The prayer of Jabez is one of my favourite prayers.

*And Jabez called on the God of Israel saying, "Oh, that You would bless me indeed, and enlarge my territory, that Your hand would be with me, and that You would keep me from evil, that I may not cause pain." So God granted him what he requested.* (1 Chronicles 4:10, NKJV)

My prayer is that He will continue to enlarge my territory, even when I am incapacitated. With ALS it is likely that my own body will become my prison.

I also love the poem, "To Althea, from Prison" by Richard Lovelace, 1642: "Stone walls do not a prison make, / Nor iron bars a cage; / Minds innocent and quiet take / That for a hermitage."

I'm making a list of what I will take with me into my seclusion. I will not be alone because the Lord has promised to go with me, just the two of us. He will shepherd me through that experience. He will make me lay down in green pastures. He will anoint my head with oil. I will fear no evil. He will be with me through the valley of the shadow of death, even through death itself.

Since there will come a time when God will be with you in your seclusion, be sure you recognize His voice. Because He *will* be talking to you.

## CHAPTER SIXTEEN

# Hearing God's Voice

There is a difference between hearing God's voice and hearing the Word of God. First let's look at familiar Bible characters who heard God's voice. Adam and Eve heard God speak to them in the garden: "*Then the Lord God called to the man, 'Where are you?'*" (Genesis 3:9, NLT). God spoke to Moses from the burning bush. God spoke to Hagar, Rahab, Simeon, Joseph, Mary, and Paul on the road to Damascus.

People hear the Lord's voice in different ways. Samuel, as a young boy, heard the Lord speak to him in an audible voice (1 Samuel 3:10). After the windstorm, earthquake, and thunder, Elijah, in 1 Kings 19:12 heard a still, small voice. "*My sheep hear my voice, and I know them, and they follow me,*" Jesus says in John 10:27, NKJV. Sometimes God's voice comes silently within us. Sometimes it's a nudge to motivate us. He might bring a person to mind over and over again; that's a good indication God wants you to visit them.

Everyone who has yielded their lives to Jesus as their saviour has heard His voice, the voice of conviction. The third verse of a hymn by James Drummond Burns, "Hushed was the Evening," is a prayer I pray often for myself: "O give me Samuel's ear, / an open ear, O Lord, alive and quick to hear / each whisper of thy word; / like him to answer to thy call, / and obey thee first of all." If this hasn't been part of your life until now, learn to tune your ear to God's voice. You'll be surprised at how often He speaks to you.

The Spirit living within us never dies. It's that part of us that goes on to live in heaven. So, when a person is totally incapacitated, when not a single muscle can move, they can still communicate with God, Spirit to spirit. A great book to get you started on this path is *Children, Can You Hear Me?: How to Hear and See God* by Brad Jersak. Begin now to fine-tune that connection.

It's common knowledge in the medical world that people who are in a coma and unresponsive hear everything that's said around them. When my father was in that state, every time a member of the family walked into the room, we watched his blood pressure rise on the monitor. A friend of mine was in a coma following a car accident.

When he came out of that coma, he knew that God had been communicating with him, that heaven was real, and that he had to share his experience with others.

That is a word of warning. Be careful what you say at the bedside of an unresponsive person. They are listening and so is the Lord.

## CHAPTER SEVENTEEN
*Your Scripture Alphabet*

The mother of a friend of mine had many long silent nights in a senior's home, but she had prepared well. She memorized scripture verses beginning with every letter of the alphabet. You can do that too. Start with uplifting verses you know.

Here is my Scripture alphabet.

"...**A**ll things are possible to him who believes." (Mark 9:23, NLT)

"**B**lessed are the merciful: for they shall obtain mercy." (Matthew 5:7)

"**C**ome unto me, all ye that labour and are heavy laden, and I will give you rest." (Matthew 11:28)

"**D**o not withhold good from those who deserve it..." (Proverbs 3:27, NLT)

"**E**very good gift and every perfect gift is from above..." (James 1:17, NKJV)

"**F**inally, be ye all of one mind, having compassion one of another..." (1 Peter 3:8)

"**G**reat is the Lord, and greatly to be praised..." (Psalm 48:1)

"**H**e is not here: for he is risen, as he said. Come, see the place where the Lord lay." (Matthew 28:6)

"**I** have written your name on the palms of my hands..." (Isaiah 49:16, NLT)

"**J**oyful are the people of integrity, who follow the instructions of the Lord." (Psalm 119:1, NLT)

"...**K**nock, and it will be opened to you." (Matthew 7:7, NKJV)

"**L**et me proclaim... your mighty miracles to all who come after me." (Psalm 71:18, NLT)

"**M**ake thankfulness your sacrifice to God." (Psalm 50:14, NLT).

"**N**arrow is the way, which leadeth unto life, and few there be that find it." (Matthew 7:14)

"**O** praise the Lord, all ye nations: praise Him, all ye people." (Psalm 117:1)

"...**P**erfect love casteth out fear..." (1 John 4:18)

"**Q**uench not the Spirit." (1 Thessalonians 5:19)

"**R**emember, O Lord, thy tender mercies and thy lovingkindnesses..." (Psalm 25:6)

"**S**o we don't look at the troubles we can see now; rather, we fix our gaze on things that cannot be seen..." (2 Corinthians 4:18, NKJV)

"**T**ruly my soul waiteth upon God: from him cometh my salvation." (Psalm 62:1)

"**U**nderstanding is a wellspring of life onto him who hath it..." (Proverbs 16:22)

"...**V**engeance is mine; I will repay, saith the Lord." (Romans 12:19)

"**W**ithhold not thou thy tender mercies from me, O Lord..." (Psalm 40:11)

**X** is the symbol for Christ—our everything.

"**Y**e also, as lively stones, are built up a spiritual house, an holy priesthood..." (1 Peter 2:5)

"...**Z**eal of the Lord of hosts will perform this." (Isaiah 9:7)

## Chapter Eighteen
# In God's Time, for God's Glory

The Holy Spirit can communicate with our spirit, even when no part of our body works. If you have a friend or a loved one with dementia, ask the Holy Spirit to bypass the physical and mental disabilities and commune with them, Spirit to spirit. Pray for that to be a daily thing in their lives. He can do that for us, and Scripture tell us it will be healing for your body and strength for your bones (Proverbs 3:7–8, NLT).

Think of the unlimited prayer ministry you can carry on, even when you are unable to communicate with people around you. God still hears you, and God still speaks to others. Who's to say you won't still be an instrument of

God's hand? Nothing can stop you from waging spiritual warfare on behalf of others. Those of us with ALS need to prepare ourselves for that season of our lives.

The seventeenth chapter of the Gospel of John gives us an amazing view into the prayer life of Jesus. In John 17:20–21 Jesus says:

> *Neither do I pray for these alone, but for them also which shall believe on me through their word; that they all may be one; as thou, Father, art in me, and I in thee, that they also may be one in us; that the world may believe that thou hast sent me.*

That sounds like we too, can be praying for those yet to be saved.

Psalm 139:17–18 the Psalmist writes: "*How precious also are thy thoughts unto me, O God! How great is the sum of them! If I should count them, they are more in number than the sand: when I awake, I am still with thee.*" When you think of God, He is thinking of you. What a comfort to know that.

Hebrews 12:1–2 are well-known verses:

> *Wherefore seeing we also are compassed about with so great a cloud of witnesses, let us lay aside every weight.... Looking unto Jesus the author and finisher of our faith; who for the joy that was set before him endured the cross, despising the shame, and is set down at the right hand of the throne of God.*

Even in our eventual solitude, there will be a great cloud of witnesses encouraging us, as well as the Lord.

We know that:

> ...*The Spirit also helpeth our infirmities: for we know not what we should pray for as we ought: but the Spirit itself maketh intercession for us with groaning which cannot be uttered. And he that searcheth the hearts knoweth what is the mind of the Spirit, because he maketh intercession for the saints according to the will of God.* (Romans 8:26–27)

Isn't that an amazing thought, that while we pray for others, the Spirit is praying for us?

So prepare to be an intercessor by praying for family, friends, medical staff, and everyone the Lord brings to your mind. Find comfort in knowing the Holy Spirit is interceding for you.

## CHAPTER NINETEEN

# Available Care

Home care, palliative care, and hospice are all available to people with chronic, long term illnesses. Home care helps people live independently in the community in their own homes. It is delivered by health care professionals, nurses, volunteers, friends, and family. Home care often depends on what the family can or can't provide.

Provincial, territorial and/or municipal governments fund home care. It is not insured through the Canada Health Act, but is funded through transfer payments for health and social services. The federal government also provides funding for home care to First Nations on-reserve,

Inuit in designated communities, members of the armed forces, RCMP, federal inmates, and eligible veterans.

Home care helps with bathing, dressing, and feeding, but it can also provide physiotherapy, occupational, and speech therapy, social work, dietitian services, homemaking, and respite services. Home care workers have special training and expertise in pain management and symptom control. They specialize in helping patients and their families cope with the many burdens of a serious illness, from the side effects of a medical treatment, to caregiver stress, to fears about the future. They can assist you with difficult medical decisions and help you weigh the pros and cons of various treatments.

Another aspect of senior care is short-term respite care. It is designed to give family caregivers a break to attend to their own needs, or during times of mental and physical exhaustion. Specific beds are designated in care homes for these situations. Check out Community Care Access Centres in your area. Those centres are local organizations established by the Ministry of Health and Long-term Care and help people access government-funded home and community services, and long-term care homes.

Shortly after my diagnosis, someone suggested to me that I should put myself on palliative care. I knew nothing about palliative care, but I have since discovered it is designed to make life more comfortable when one has a serious, life-threatening or chronic illness, and it can begin as soon as one is diagnosed. It focuses on improving a patient's quality of life, including pain management, speech therapy, and emotional care. Palliative care may also involve physical, spiritual, emotional, or legal assistance. At the end of life, palliative care may be the only treatment available.

Palliative care is care of the whole person that relieves the symptoms of a disease whether or not it can be cured. Hospice, on the other hand, is a specific type of palliative care for people who are near end of life.

Palliative doctors have specialized in palliative medicine, concentrating on preventing and alleviating suffering, improving your quality of life, and helping you and your loved ones cope with the stress and burden of your illness. A palliative care team may include a nurse, pharmacist, social worker, dietitian, and volunteers, and can be provided at a hospital, a nursing home, an assisted-living facility, or at home with necessary equipment, such as a hospital bed, brought in.

Healthcare is a shared jurisdiction in Canada. Delivery of healthcare is primarily the responsibility of provincial and territorial governments. Under the Canada Health Act, the federal government provides financial support to provinces and territories, but they are also responsible for funding and/or delivering care to certain populations. It is not surprising that care, including palliative care, differs significantly across the country, due to our vast and diverse geography, demographics and shared jurisdictions.

The Canadian health system is often thought of as being universal and comprehensive, but only hospital services that are medically necessary, as defined by each province/territory, are currently insured under the Canada Health Act. Additional care and services may be paid for in whole or part by provincial policies, private insurers, or by patients and families themselves. This complex and piecemeal funding is particularly problematic for palliative care, since it can be delivered outside a hospital setting.

Improving access to hospice palliative care through community integration is a goal that has been identified by leaders across Canada: The Quality End-of Life Care Coalition of Canada, the Canadian Hospice Palliative Care Association, and the Canadian Frailty Network.

End of life care is constantly being assessed by private and government groups.

## Chapter Twenty
### *Waiting on the Lord*

In spite of doing so well for so many years with ALS, I know I will die someday and I pray that when the time is right, I will *die well*. I am sure some of you reading this book have reached your place of solitude before me. Perhaps, right now, you are secluded with the Lord, with no ability to interact with people around you.

I would like to pray for you right now. *May God's presence be manifested with you. I pray that the Lord will commune with you, Spirit to spirit. I pray that the scriptures you have learned in the past will quicken in your heart, to be health to your heart and strength to your bones. I pray the Lord will give you patience to wait on the Lord's timing. Amen.*

A Christian doctor told me once about being at the bedsides of Christians when they left this life. "It is a beautiful experience," he told me with awe in his voice. "If you watch close, you can sense the moment the spirit departs." How much closer can we get to glory than at that moment?

Waiting was a huge part of Jesus' life. He waited until after Lazarus died to arrive at their house, but what an amazing outcome. He raised Lazarus from the dead.

People have suggested I have ALS because of things I have done, an attack of the enemy, or for my discipline, but not once has anyone suggested that it might be so that the works of God would be revealed in me. We always want someone or something to blame. We'd rather turn away from difficult questions and avoid controversy. I have yielded my life to the Lord so that He would be glorified. Would He even allow something like ALS if He wasn't going to receive glory in the long-run? My life is in His hands.

## CHAPTER TWENTY-ONE
## Embrace Eternity

*Eternity* is defined as what exists outside of time. While we live on earth, we live in time; we have a beginning and an end. God, on the other hand is eternal; He had no beginning and no end. It's an interesting thought, that when we die, we will be eternal, even though we had a beginning.

What would have happened if Adam and Eve had not eaten of the tree of knowledge of good and evil, the only tree they were told *not* to eat of? The tree of life was not forbidden. What a different story if they had eaten of the Tree of Life first. After they made the wrong choice, sin entered their hearts and God sent them out of the garden so they could not eat of the tree of life and live forever in their sin Then, He set a guard around the Tree of Life (Genesis 3:22–24).

But God set in place an amazing plan to redeem humanity from sin. When we partake in His plan, we will live with Him eternally, without sin, and The Tree of Life is available to us in heaven. If you have never accepted His sacrifice to pay for your sins, do it now. Thank Him for dying in your place and tell Him that you want to be His child. A miracle will take place in your heart and mind.

You often see John 3:16 written on signs at sporting events. I'm sure it is the most quoted verse in the Bible: "*For God so loved the world that He gave His only begotten son, that whosoever believes in Him shall not perish but have eternal life.*" Eternity with God was His plan for us from the very beginning.

In John 17:5, Jesus must have been longing to return to the Father when He prayed, *And now, O Father glorify thou me with... the glory I had with thee before the world was.*" Our finite minds find it difficult to think of Jesus living in Glory with the Father before the world (and time) began. Our image of before creation is the earth, formless and void, with darkness hovering over the face of the water. But God was there, so it must have been bright and glorious.

But that was before God created our world as we know it. We have the creation story well-learned, and we know we are here on earth to be ambassadors for Christ.

How are we doing? Do we so enjoy being ambassadors that we really don't want to leave this world? Let's be honest. This life is one of sickness and pain, sorrow, and depression. It's time to look at the other side of the story.

Jesus told the disciples He was going to prepare a place for them: "*And if I go and prepare a place for you, I will come again, and receive you unto myself; that where I am, there ye may be also*" (John 14:3).

The goal of palliative care is to provide comfort, and help each of us *die well,* but it is up to each one of us to be prepared. Medications are available so no one has to die in pain. Make sure you have a living will in place and advanced directives shared with family, doctor, and clergy. You can choose your own environment for the last days and hours of your human life.

## CHAPTER TWENTY-TWO
# You are Invited to My Bedside

If you love the Word of God and are in the habit of reading His word often, think ahead to a time when you may not have the strength to hold a Bible or turn the pages. Prepare now. Purchase the Bible on CD that you can listen to. Try it out and make sure you like the sound of the reader's voice. With that also comes the need to have a CD player and maybe even headphones.

Don't be embarrassed by what you can and can't do, or what you look like. God loves what He sees when He sees you. When the disease has progressed, you will appreciate visits from friends and family, bringing community, church, and world news to you. They will see your spirit shining out of you. Invite your small group to meet in your room and listen to the podcast of the Sunday service together. Have friends load your iPod with your favourite songs.

God will still speak to you and you will still talk to Him. You will remember the scriptures you have learned. You will sense God's presence with you. You will welcome people speaking about the Lord, and maybe someone else nearby will be blessed, too. In that way, too, you will glorify the Lord.

But for right now, smile. People expect us to be discouraged and sad. Smile, and people will see Christ in your life. Caregivers love patients who have the love of Christ flowing through them. If you are filled with the love of Christ, His love flowing through you will minister to those who assist you.

Christ identifies with us. He left His place in heaven to be born as a baby, totally helpless, unable to talk, walk, speak, and needing total care. He understands what you are going through. He left the glories of Heaven willingly, so He could purchase eternal life for us through the shedding of His blood.

Now, we have the option to glorify Him in our bodies: *"That is why we never give up. Though our bodies are dying, our spirits are being renewed every day"* (2 Corinthians 4:16, NLT).

I have designed a poster to be put on the wall beside my bed.

Family, friends, staff,
I have ALS.
I can't respond to you
because my muscles don't work,
but my brain is alert
and functioning.
I hear what you say.
I still talk to God.
Tell me your prayer requests.
I will take them to the
throne of God for you.

## CHAPTER TWENTY-THREE
### The Sacrifice of Praise

What is the sacrifice of praise? It's a willing offering of praise to the Lord, giving thanks in every situation, especially in difficult times.

I remember my grandpa living with us in a house so tiny I don't even know where he slept. He was a kind, loving man, but he wasn't well. When we had a meal, he had only bread soaked in milk. One day, I set up a lemonade stand in front of our house. Grandpa often sat in a lawn chair in the back yard, soaking up the sun. I asked grandpa if he would buy a glass of lemonade. He did.

It broke my heart when he died from stomach cancer months later. I loved him and he loved me. He was an alcoholic all his life, and my own father lived through that; he saw his parents separate and the family fall apart.

Yet my father took my grandpa into our home and cared for him. My father demonstrated the power of love and forgiveness. Today, I can praise the Lord for what I learned about love from those two men. Grandpa paid for a glass of lemonade he couldn't drink. He secretly poured his lemonade on the ground because he loved me.

We often forget that Christ had such great love for us, that He died for us when we were still in our sin. Could any situation be so profound that we can't praise the Lord? As Psalm 22:3 says, "*You are holy, enthroned on the praises of Israel.*"

Hebrews 13:14–15 says, "*This world is not our permanent home; we are looking forward to a home yet to come. Therefore let us offer through Jesus a continual sacrifice of praise to God, proclaiming our allegiance to his name*" (NLT). Even now, when ALS has invaded our lives, we are still told to bring an offering (sacrifice) of praise to the Lord. Thank you, Lord, for dying for me. Thank you, Lord, for your great love. Thank you, Lord, for eternal life that awaits me.

When Job learned his entire family had been killed, he said, "*I came naked from my mother's womb, and I will be naked when I leave. The Lord gave me what I had and the Lord has taken it away. Praise the name of the Lord!*" (Job 1:21, NLT). Verse 22 continues: "*In all of this, Job did not sin by blaming God.*"

Remember the promise of Romans 8:22–23, NLT:

*For we know that all creation has been groaning as in the pains of childbirth right up to the present time. And we believers also groan, even though we have the Holy Spirit within us as a foretaste of future glory, for we long for our bodies to be released from sin and suffering. We too, wait with eager hope for the day when God will give us our full rights as his adopted children, including the new bodies he has promised us.*

CHAPTER TWENTY-FOUR
# At Home with the Father

As the years pass by, I find myself thinking more and more about heaven and being with the Lord. I am excited when I think that my knees will bow before Him. I'll have strength to lift my hands in praise to Him. I'll sing again and speak again. The following verses I share with you because they have brought peace into my life.

> *I am overwhelmed with joy in the Lord my God! For he has dressed me with the clothing of salvation and draped me in a robe of righteousness. I am like a bridegroom in his wedding suit or a bride with her jewels.* (Isaiah 61:10, NLT)

*And God will wipe away every tear from their eyes; there shall be no more death, nor sorrow, nor crying. There shall be no more death, neither shall there be any more pain, for the former things have passed away.* (Revelation 21:4, NKJV)

*And he said unto me, "It is done. I am Alpha and Omega, the beginning and the end. I will give onto him that is athirst of the fount of the water of life freely. He that overcometh shall inherit all things; and I will be his God, and he shall be my son."* (Revelation 21:6–7)

*I saw no temple in the city, for the Lord God Almighty and the Lamb are its temple. And the city has no need of the sun or moon, for the glory of God illuminates the city, and the Lamb is its light.* (Revelation 21:22–23, NLT)

*Then the angel showed me a river with the water of life, clear as crystal, flowing from the throne of God and of the Lamb. It flowed down the center of the main street. On each side of the river grew a tree of life, bearing twelve crops of fruit, with a fresh crop each month. The leaves were used for medicine to heal the nations.* (Revelation 22:1–2, NLT)

*I, John, am the one who heard and saw all those things. And when I heard and saw them, I fell down to worship at the feet of the angel who showed them to me. But he said, "No, don't worship me, I am a servant of God, just like you and your brothers the prophets, as well as all who obey what is written in this book. Worship only God."* (Revelation 22:8–9, NLT)

*Let us be glad and rejoice, and give honour to him; for the marriage of the Lamb is come, and his wife has made herself ready. And to her was granted that she should be arrayed in fine linen, clean and white for the fine linen is the righteousness of saints.* (Revelation 19:7–8, NKJV)

*Yea, though I walk through the valley of the shadow of death, I will fear no evil: for thou art with me; thy rod and thy staff they comfort me... Thou anointest my head with oil; my cup runneth over. Surely goodness and mercy shall follow me all the days of my life: and I will dwell in the house of the Lord forever.* (Psalm 23:4–6)